NATURAL WAYS TO STAY HEALTHY

HERBAL ANTIBIOTICS FOR TREATMENT OF BACTERIA INFECTIONS

CLIFF JOHN

The information offered here is for the purposes of information only and is universal as such. The information presented here is without any form of contract or guarantee or indemnity whether with the reader or any third party.

CHAPTER ONE

Antibiotics are medications that help to stop infections in our body that are caused by bacteria. Bacteria are the main causes of infections and antibiotics helps by killing the bacteria or by stopping them from reproducing within our system. The name 'antibiotics' means 'against life' and any drugs that kills germs within our body. Antibiotics are not effective against viral infections such as flu, sore throats, common cold and most coughs.

Antibiotics are mainly used to stop or kill the growth of bacteria in our body system. Although, many has thought that antibiotics as drug is a modern medicine, this is not true because antibiotics have been around for many centuries now and the antibiotics drugs as we have it today are derived from herbal sources.

Some herbs can be antibiotics. A little sampling of about 58 Chinese plants discovered that 23 of them had antibacterial properties and another 15 of them had antifungal properties. A study in 2014 showed that herbal therapy was just as effective as a chemical antibiotics for effectiveness in the treatments of small intestine bacteria overgrowth disorder.

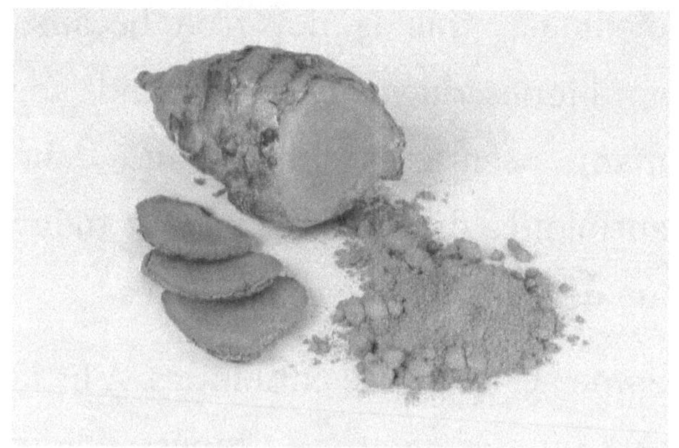

Turmeric plants are cultivated and grown in Philippines, South Asia, Taiwan, South China, and Indonesia. This plant grows very well on a good ground irrigation system where there is much rainfall. For Turmeric to produce larger rhizomes, then it will work in the tropics and sub-tropics.

Turmeric contains substance known as curcumin and this is used precisely as a refreshing tonic and to improve the body stamina so that it will not easily get tired. A study in Singapore shows that the curcumin substance in turmeric, apart from it functions as anti-Alzheimer, it can also works as a means in treating various kinds of diseases. The reason for this, is because curcumin contains several compounds such as anti-oxidant, anti-tumor promoter, anti-microbial, anti-virus and anti-inflammatory. Curcumin in turmeric also plays a role of boosting the immune system.

WHAT YOU BENEFIT FROM TURMERIC

There are several benefits health that has been attributed to turmeric and some of these health benefits are:

1. Lose Weight Treatments

Several researches has already shown the benefits of turmeric for lose weight. Developing countries and all around the world today, the excess fat of body or obesity is an emerging epidemic. The imbalance and excess of nutrient consumptions are related to the prevailing lifestyle obtainable this days and there is the needs to be concerned given to the increasing numbers of people suffering from obesity and overweight. Constant intakes of the herbal of turmeric can shrink the acid in your stomach and decrease the weight. If you desire to have a good diet without facing difficulty and taking expensive medication, just consume the turmeric acid herbal.

Abdominal fat, weight gain and obesity can be reduced in several ways, and ones of way is the anti-inflammatory and antioxidant consumption of supplements that can be gotten from various sources such as curcumin. Curcuminoid are contained in turmeric which consists of curcumin I, II and III. Also, essential oils play a significant role in weight loss and in turmeric extract there are about 25 essential oil compounds that can be found.

Curcumin is a component of phytochemicals found in turmeric. Given to its color, curcumin has been used in the food and the apparel industry. That is not all, curcumin has also been used as a traditional medicine, additional foodstuffs, and preservative in several countries.

2. Treating Typhoid and Heartburn

Turmeric substances are rich and beneficial in several ways, these includes the healing of wounds in the stomach and to treats typhoid. Use the following steps; get ready 2 turmeric, 1 sheet of bitter leaf, and 1 hump sere. After which you puree all your ingredients and boil with 1 cup of water and drink every day for one week.

3. Turmeric For Dysmenorrhea

Several researches and medical experiments has proven the health benefits of turmeric for the treatment of dysmenorrhea. On a general note, dysmenorrhea is the name given to a painful menstruation in ladies and this pains are not related to pathological abnormalities. This could be in form of; primary dysmenorrhea that occurs in the absence of pathology or the second dysmenorrhea that is as a result of identifiable organic disease. In most cases, teenage girls or younger women tends to feel more pain when it comes to primary dysmenorrhea because the hormonal cycle is very not stable. Given to this, primary dysmenorrhea has greatly disturb the activity and concentration of the sufferers.

When you experience the complaints of primary dysmenorrhea, there are several other things that you can do to help ameliorate the condition such as consume analgesic, acupuncture, compress your stomach with warm water, take physical exercise regularly, and also the constant intakes of turmeric acid can help to resolve the complaints of primary dysmenorrhea in teenager girls or young women.

4. Reducing the Risk of Alzheimer's Disease

The disease caused by inflammation of the brain is called Alzheimer. Studies has shown that persons that consume turmeric regularly have a lower chances of developing

Alzheimer's disease. This is because turmeric has the capacity to protect the brain from any form of inflammation.

5. Reducing the Risk of Diabetes

There are pathogens responsible for diabetes type 1 such as Coxsackie B4 virus and this can be prevented by the Antiviral, anti-bacterial, and antibiotics of turmeric. Turmeric contained curcumin which is very important in overcoming the insulin resistance within the body, this is given to fact the insulin resistance glucose in the blood can be controlled or regulated. With this, the risk of type 2 diabetes can be averted. Turmeric automatically prevents diabetes by controlling weight through the substance of curcumin. On how to use turmeric as diabetes treatment; get ready 3 turmerics plus ½ teaspoon of salt, 1 liter of water and boil together, make sure you strain it and drink 2 times a week, minimum ½ cup.

6. Overcoming Joints Inflammation

The curcumin substance in turmeric is also useful for anti-inflammation and this very useful for those people who suffer from arthritis and can be taken as medicine. Turmeric may be consumed as a traditional herbal medicine or it can be taken in form of modern capsule medicine.

7. Eliminating Bad Cholesterol (LDL) in the Body

Bad cholesterol can be very dangerous for our body when they are not eliminated. This bad cholesterol can result to various diseases such as narrowing of the arteries, heart disease, inflammation of the blood vessels, and other cholesterol. The nutritional content of turmeric is believed to overcome the bad cholesterol that finds their ways into the body. This however, will help to reduce the danger of diseases due to cholesterol.

8. Lowering Blood Pressure

Turmeric can also be used to reduce blood pressure, the things required are;

Ingredients

300 cc honey

Gotu kola's leaves, 50 grams

500 cc of water

3 rhizomes of fresh turmeric

Directions

Chopped into the small pieces your turmeric and Gotu kola's leaves

Mix ingredients together and boiled in 500 cc of water until you are left with 150 cc of water.

Allow it to gets cold before you drink.

Take 1 tablespoon 3 times daily.

9. Turmeric is a Stamina Booster

Turmeric has been known to increase stamina, and this can be achieved using the following ways;

Squeeze your turmeric until the water gotten fills 1 tablespoon.

Prepare 1 chicken egg, pepper powder, 1 tablespoon lemon juice, and 1 tablespoon of honey.

Add all your ingredients to a glass and stir very well until it is well coated together, wait for a minute, then

Consuming this herbal 3 times daily will help to increase your vitality.

10. Turmeric Eliminate Body Odor from the Inside

You can use turmeric to eliminated body odor, this can be achieved using the following ingredients and directions:

Grate 2 segments of fresh turmeric.

Mixed it with palm sugar in 2/3 cup of warm boiled water.

Stir very well for few minutes and then strain

Drink it once a day before you go to bed.

11. Turmeric Reduces Heat Fever

Turmeric can be very useful when you get fever, to prepare, use the following ingredients and directions:

20 grams of grated fresh turmeric.

Add in 100 ml of boiled water and stir gently until it is dissolved.

Strain your turmeric liquid

Squeeze it well to get the water out

Drink the turmeric juice in the warm temperatures.

12. Malaria Treatments

Turmeric can be used for the treatment of malaria disease using the following ingredients:

6 grams of Jering antan's leaves

3 grams of turmeric

20 grams of ginger

15 grams of skin pule

5 grams of bark keningar

500 cc of boiled water

5 grams of sandalwood

6 drops eucalyptus oil and

Directions

Blend all your ingredients together except eucalyptus oil

Boiled in 500 cc of water.

Drink the herbal when it gets cold for 3 times daily.

13.   Turmeric   For   Diarrhoea Treatment

Turmeric can be used for the treatment of diarrhoea disease using the following <u>Ingredients</u>:

Ingredients:

Piece of ules of wood,

3 coriander seeds

 Alum leaves,

½ penetrance angina.

½ finger turmeric.

Directions:

Mix all your ingredients together

Boiled them in 150 ml water

Strain your boiling water, and drink the herb when it is ready {please allow to cool}.

Consume it morning and evening, taking 75 ml each.

14. Late Periods

Turmeric can also be used for the treatment of late period in woman using the following ingredients:

Ingredients

15 grams of Sigading's leaves

Turmeric

10 grams of cardamom

Nutmeg

5 grams of black cumin

Coriander, and cloves

Directions

Boil in 3 cups of water all ingredients and wait for water to boil remaining 1 cup.

Strain the water and taking medication1/3 cup 3 times daily.

12. Menstruation is not Smooth

Turmeric can also be used for the treatment of menstruation related issues in woman using the following <u>Ingredients</u>:

Coriander ½ tea spoon

Turmeric,

½ tea spoon of Nutmeg

½ handful of leaves spreading.

Directions:

Mixed all ingredients together, finely and boiled with 1 liter of water,

Strain and drink one cup per day.

15. Appendix

Turmeric can also be used for the treatment of appendix using the following ingredients:

1 turmeric

1 whole lemon

1 slice of coconut sugar/palm

Salt to taste.

Directions:

Grated your turmeric and squeezed the lime juice

Mixed it with other ingredients and brewed with 1 cup of hot water, after which you filtered.

Drink it every morning after having breakfast.

17. Turmeric Helps Prevent Heartburn

Turmeric can also be used for the prevention of heartburn using the following ingredients:

How to use:

Take 1 seed of medium size turmeric, and cleaned it.

Grated your turmeric into small portions and keep one aside.

Add brown sugar as the flavour and mix them together in the hot water.

Keep stirring until it appears thickened.

Strain and drink it while it is still warm.

<u>Making Turmeric Acid Herbal</u>

Instructions

Prepare and mashed 1 piece of turmeric

Boil 2 cups of water

Add the juice of tamarind and brown sugar to create a better taste.

Cook mixture into half or one glass.

Drink it either in cold or warm.

CHAPTER TWO

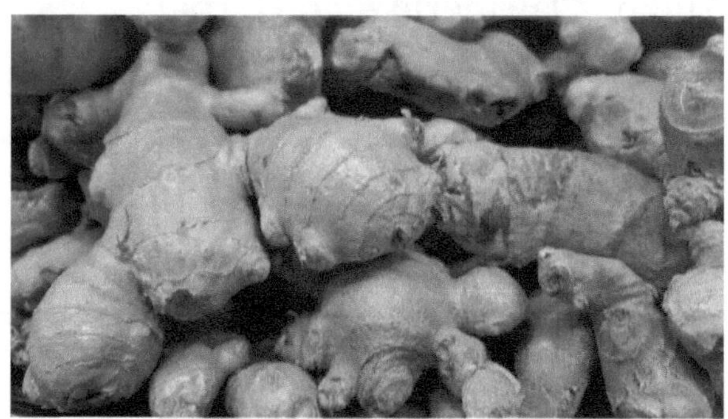

Ginger belongs to the Zingiberaceae family, and it is closely related to cardamom, turmeric, and galangal. It is one of the healthiest and most delicious cooking spices that you can find on the planet earth. Ginger is loaded with lots of nutrients and bioactive compounds that have powerful benefits for the brain and body.

Ginger can be found in capsules, fresh or ginger essential oil and the health benefits are well known and has been used globally as a natural solutions for thousands of years because of its medicinal properties. It has been recorded that ancient Greek, Chinese, Arabic and Romans have all been identified with the health benefits of ginger root for well-being.

There are many important vitamins and minerals that are present inside ginger. There is gingerol, that is, a compound with potent anti-inflammatory and antioxidant. And has many health benefits. A fresh and raw ginger approximately contains the following

17.8 grams of carbohydrates

80 calories

1.8 grams of protein

415 milligrams of potassium

0.7 grams of fat

0.2 milligrams of copper

2 grams of dietary

43 milligrams of manganese

34 milligrams of phosphorus

Also, ginger contains other nutrients outside the above listed nutrients such as zinc, calcium, thiamine, pantothenic acid and riboflavin.

WHAT GINGER ADDS TO YOU

1. Ginger Protects Against Stomach Ulcers

These are painful sores that are formed in the lining of our stomach and usually have the symptoms of fatigue, indigestion, abdominal discomfort and heartburn.

Several researches have shown that ginger goes a long way to help prevent the formation of stomach ulcers. In 2011, research on an animal found that ginger powder protected against aspirin-induced stomach ulcers and this is done by decreasing levels of inflammatory proteins in the body and also blocking the activity of ulcer causing enzymes.

2. Ginger Helps Treat Nausea

Right from time immemorial ginger has been used as a natural remedy for morning sickness, sea sickness and it is also perhaps well-known for its ability to treat vomiting and nausea.

A results of 12 studies that comprises of 1,278 pregnant women and shown that ginger was very effective at decreasing the symptoms of nausea with very minimal side effects. Also, another research from the University of Rochester Medical Center proved that ginger has helped to reduce nausea severity in patients receiving chemotherapy.

3. Ginger Eases Menstrual Pains

Menstruation for many women are commonly accompanied with many side effects like period cramps (dysmenorrhea) headaches, and pain.

While some medications provides some symptoms relief, some natural remedies like ginger can be very useful when it comes to easing menstrual pain.

A research that was published in the Journal of Alternative and Complementary Medicine found that ginger reduces menstrual pain as effectively as other medications like mefanamic acid and ibuprofen. Similarly another research in 2009 reported that ginger reduces both the intensity and duration of pain menstrual.

4. Ginger Helps Fights Fungal Infections

There are variety of conditions that causes fungal infections, and these ranges from yeast infections to jock itch and athlete's foot. Given to its powerful anti-fungal properties, ginger helps kill off disease-causing fungi.

With a test-tube study carried out in Iran 2016, it was discovered that ginger extract are very effective against two major types of yeast which are common causes of fungal infections in the mouth. Similarly, a test-tube research in Mycoses to measure the antifungal effects of 29 different plant species discovered that ginger was the most effective of them all at killing off fungus.

5. Ginger Helps Inhibit Cancer Growth

Another powerful benefits of ginger is its anti-cancer properties, this is as a result of the presence of a very powerful compound known as 6-gingerol.

A Test-tube research found that ginger and its components can be very effective in blocking cancer cell growth and development for prostate cancer, ovarian and pancreatic. There is however, need for more research to determine as to how the properties of ginger may inhibits cancer and how it translate to humans.

6. Ginger Helps Improves Brain Function

Neurodegenerative conditions such as Parkinson's and Alzheimer's disease have been directly linked to oxidative stress and chronic inflammation in the brain. Ginger with her valuable antioxidants and potent anti-inflammatory properties, it is believed to play an important role in brain health.

Different animal researches have shown that ginger extract could guide against brain aging and cognitive decline. That is not all, a 2012 study also showed that ginger extract helped improve attention and cognitive function in middle-aged women.

7. Ginger Helps Regulates Blood Sugar

There are many negative symptoms attributed to high blood sugar in the body, these ranges from constant urination to increased thirst and headaches (including migraines). When these are not properly cater for, it can result to a more serious problems like the damage of the nerve and impaired wound healing.

Studies has found that ginger helps to normalise blood sugar level in order to prevent these serious side effects. In a 2015 research, it was found that ginger supplementation actually reduced fasting blood sugar level by 12 percent and also improved long-term blood sugar control by 10 percent.

8. Ginger Helps Blocks Bacterial Infections

Apart from ginger's antifungal properties, it's also boasts the ability to fight off bacterial infections in the body. Pathogens responsible for bacteria are common culprits behind conditions like bronchitis, urinary tract infections and pneumonia.

According to a test-tube research, the compounds present in ginger could help stop the growth of certain ancestry of bacteria that cause gum disease. Similarly, another test-tube research found that ginger extract was very effective against several types of drug-resistant bacteria as well.

9. Ginger Helps Promotes Proper Digestion

Another powerful benefits of ginger is its ability to support digestive health and prevent health challenge like dyspepsia, a frequent condition of an impaired digestion mostly characterized by symptoms like heartburn, pain, discomfort and fullness.

A study in the World Journal of Gastroenterology, shows that ginger helps to speed up the emptying of the stomach by 25 percent when compared to a placebo in people with digestion related problems. Similarly, another study also found that consuming ginger capsules with a meal actually increase the speed of stomach emptying.

10. Ginger Helps Relieves Joint and Muscle Pain

With ginger's ability to reduce inflammation, adding it to your diet can help treat both arthritis-related joint pain and muscle pain.

Research has found that daily intakes of ginger resulted in moderate to large reductions in muscle pain which could be caused by exercise-induced muscle injury. Similarly, another study also found that ginger extract helps to decrease knee pain and the need for pain medication in individuals with osteoarthritis.

11. Ginger Helps Eases Inflammation

Some inflammation could be a normal, healthy immune response to infection and injury, but chronic inflammation is found to be a major contributor to related issues like cancer, heart disease, diabetes and obesity.

A review in International Journal of Preventive Medicine noted that ginger extract could help stop the synthesis of certain inflammation markers. Apart from gingerol, ginger also contains other anti-inflammatory compounds like zingerone, shogaol, and paradol.

CHAPTER THREE

NEVER FORGET THIS ONE

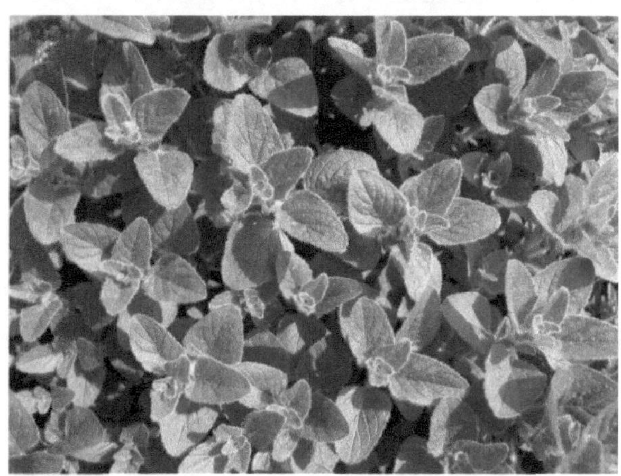

Oregano plant

Oregano plant is a fragrant herb that normally used to flavor pasta and meat dishes, and they is known for their universality in the kitchen. This plant can however be transformed into an herbal oil that is embedded with several benefits. Oregano oil is however gotten from the leaves and flowers of the oregano plants, which is a hardy perennial herb, and belong to the mint family. It's can be found in Asia, Europe, North Africa and other parts of the world.

As a perennial plant, oregano can grows up to 50 centimetres high, and has a purple leaves that are between 2 - 3 centimetres long. The name oregano comes from two Greek words which "oros" meaning 'mountain' and "ganos," meaning 'joy' which when joined together, oregano literally means "joy of the mountain." This wonderful plant has been deeply appreciated by the ancient Greeks and Romans, using it for various medicinal purposes.

Oregano has been revered to as a symbol of happiness, and in the ancient world it was tradition to crown brides and grooms with a laurel of oregano. Oregano has over 40 species, but the most beneficial to health is the oil that is produced from wild oregano which is dominant in the Mediterranean regions. This essential oil from oregano is pracrically extracted through steam distillation using oregano shoots and leaves.

DO YOU HAVE OREGANO OIL?

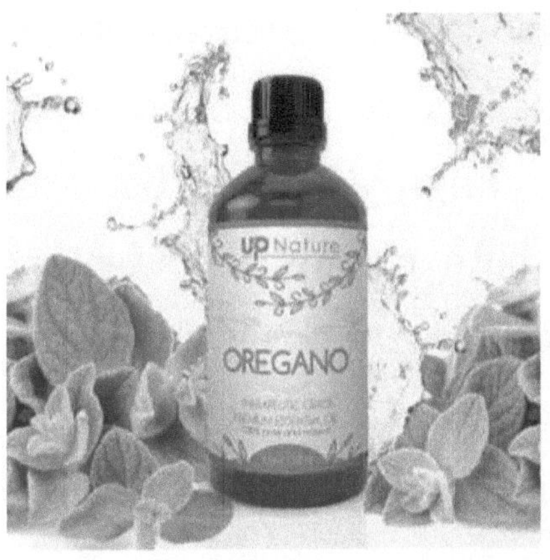

One of the most notable healing compound that can be found in an oregano oil is carvacrol, and it is with widespread of uses ranges from treatment of allergies to protecting our skin. According a research by the Faculty of Pharmacy at the University of Messina in Italy and they have this to say:

"Carvacrol, a monoterpenic phenol, has emerged for its wide spectrum activity extended to food spoilage or pathogenic fungi, yeast and bacteria as well as human, animal and plant pathogenic microorganisms including drug-resistant and biofilm forming microorganisms".

Carcavol which can be found in oregano essential oil has been referenced to as the world's No. 1 database for scientific evidence-based literature in PubMed, and has been the focus of over 800 researches. Carvacrol is multi-functional and impressive and has been shown in several researches to help reduce or reverse some of the following health related problems:

Fungal infections

Allergies

Parasites

Indigestion

Bacterial infections

Candida

Inflammation

Tumors

Viruses

Also oregano has an antimicrobial properties that helps it to preserve food quality during storage

1. Fights Infections & Bacterial Overgrowth

Researches has shown that oregano essential oil can help to fight many different group of bacteria that cause harm to our body and these bacteria are commonly treated with antibiotics. Several studies have attested to the fact that oregano oil can be used to replace many harmful antibiotics for health concerns.

The Journal of Medicinal Food {JMF} in 2011 published a research work that examined the antibacterial effects of an oregano oil when used against five different species of bad bacteria. After examining the anti-bacterial features of an oregano oil, it was discovered that there is significant anti-bacterial properties against all five types of bad bacteria. The peak of their activity was seen against E. Coli, which shows that oregano oil can potentially be used on a routine basis to prevent deadly food poisoning and to promote gastrointestinal health.

A research work published in Journal of the Science of Food and Agriculture in 2013 concluded that "Oregano extracts and essential oil from Portuguese origin are strong candidates to replace synthetic chemicals used by the industry." Experts from this research discovered that after studying the antibacterial and antioxidant properties of oregano that Origanum vulgare stops the growth of seven tested groups of bacteria which other plant extracts could not.

Also another research work involving mice which was published in the journal Revista Brasileira de Farmacognosia also discovered an impressive results which says that: apart from fighting bacteria like E. Coli and Listeria, oregano oil has also been discovered to have the ability to help pathogenic fungi.

2. Natural Alternative to Antibiotics

One of the major challenge with frequently using broad-spectrum antibiotics can be risky because broad-spectrum antibiotics do not only kill bacteria that causes infections, but also kill good bacteria that are essential for optimal health.

A fantastic article printed by the Wall Street Journal highlighted the side effects that patients may have to cope with when they use antibiotics repeatedly. In the writer's words, "Recent studies have shown that doctors are overprescribing broad-spectrum antibiotics, sometimes called the big guns that kill a wide swath of both good and bad bacteria in the body."

Too much of antibiotics, and broad-spectrum drugs prescriptions when they are not needed, can result to different health related problems. This can make the drugs to be less effective against the bacteria they are intended to treat by fostering the growth of antibiotic-resistant infections. This can in turn wipe out the good bacteria (probiotics) in body, which assist to digest food, produce vitamins and protect from infections, among many other functions.

Broad-spectrum antibiotics are commonly prescribed most often for conditions that they are not needed, for example is viral infections. In a research work published in the Journal of Antimicrobial Chemotherapy, the researchers which were from the University of Utah and the Center for Disease Control and Prevention (CDC) discovered that about 60 percent of most time when physicians prescribe antibiotics, the types they prescribed are the broad-spectrum. Similarly another research work of children, which was published in the journal Pediatrics, discovered that the antibiotics prescribed were mainly broad-spectrum.

Oil of oregano on the contrary is a "broad-spectrum approach" to protecting your health. The active ingredients of an oregano oil help to fight multiple types of harmful pathogens, including fungi, bacteria, and yeast. A research work published in the Journal of Medicinal Food journal in 2013 stated, that oregano oils "represent an inexpensive source of natural antibacterial substances that exhibited potential for use in pathogenic systems."

3. Oregano Oil Helps Treat Athlete's Foot

A research work has found that the combination of salt, heat and the use of essential oils (such as oregano) had inhibitory effects against conidia of T. mentagrophytes and mycelia of T. rubrum, group of bacteria with similar trend which are the common cause of fungal infection known as athlete's foot. This research was concluded on the note that "Thermotherapy combined with essential oils and salt would be promising to treat tinea pedis in a foot bath." Haven tested the fungicidal activity of 11 different essential oils against the bacteria that are responsible for athlete's foot, it was found that oregano oil was the most powerful (which was closely followed by cinnamon bark, thyme, clove and lemongrass).

4. Oregano Oil Helps Reduce Side Effects From Drugs/ Medications

Over the years, several research work have discovered that one of the most promising benefits of oregano oil is her ability to help reduce the side effects from drugs/ medications. These researches have given hope to persons who are looking for ways to manage the negative side effects that accompanies medical interventions and drugs, such as use of drugs for chronic conditions like arthritis or chemotherapy.

A research work that was published in the International Journal of Clinical and Experimental Medicine proved that phenol found in an oil of oregano can help to protect against methotrexate toxicity in mice. These are drugs that are commonly used to treat a wide array of issues from rheumatoid arthritis to cancer, which is also well-known to have dangerous side effects. It was concluded after evaluation that oil of oregano's has the ability to checkmate these factors, researchers believe it is due to oregano's anti-inflammatory and antioxidants properties. This wonder oil was shown to work better than drugs that are ineffective at providing full protection against methotrexate adverse effects. Through evaluation of different markers in the sciatic nerve in mice, it was discovered for the first time that carvacrol reduced the pro-inflammatory response in mice being treated by methotrexate.

In another research that was conducted in the Netherlands, it was found that oregano essential oil can also "prevent bacterial overgrowth and colonization in the large intestine during oral iron therapy." Oregano essential oil helps to treat iron deficiency anaemia and oral iron therapy known to cause a series of gastrointestinal issues like diarrhoea, vomiting, constipation, nausea and heartburn.

It has been said that carvacrol aims at the outer membrane of gram-negative bacteria and increases membrane permeability, which will result in depletion of harmful bacteria. Apart from caracole antimicrobial properties, it's also have to do with certain pathways for handling bacterial iron which helps to lower side effects of iron therapy.

5. Oregano Help in Managing Inflammatory Conditions

Whether in dry or fresh form, oregano retains its strong antioxidant capacity. Given to oregano essential oil high concentration of antioxidants its can help reduce oxidative damage and also help in preventing carcinogenesis, mutagenesis, and aging as a result of its "free radical scavenging activities." Free radicals are accepted to be a contributing factor to common chronic conditions including cardiovascular diseases, cancer, drug toxicity and neurodegenerative disorders.

One research has found that a combined treatment with oregano essential oils and thyme helped to reduce the production of pro-inflammatory cytokines, which may however help attenuate colitis in mice. Other researches also discovered that oregano oil is beneficial for treating rheumatoid arthritis, reoccurring respiratory disorders, and tumour growth. Researchers in Argentina from the Universidad Nacional de Córdoba also showed evidence that essential oil isolated from oregano "presents antibacterial, antioxidant and chemopreventive properties and could be play an important role as bioprotector agent."

6. Oregano Oil Helps Treat Digestive Issues

The active compounds in an Oregano oil can help in digestion by helping to balance the ratio of good-to-bad bacteria in the gut and also by relaxing the muscles of the GI tract. One of the active compounds of oregano's oil known as thymol, which is a similar compound found in peppermint oil known menthol. Thymol like menthol, may help to relax the soft tissue of the stomach and throat which can help to reduce GERD, discomfort and heartburn after eating.

Given to the fact it helps fights yeast overgrowth and balance bacteria, oregano essential oil is also a common natural treatment for SIBO and Candida or small intestine bacterial excessive growth. SIBO is a popular digestive problem that causes bloating, gas and intolerances to many carbohydrate-containing foods. Oregano essential oil help to stop bacterial replication and can also be used in similarity to antibiotic medications such as rifaximin for the treatment of infections that affect nutrient absorption and digestive health.

A research work published in Global Advances in Health & Medicine 2014 discovered that the use of herbal antimicrobials is very effective just like the antibiotic that is usually given for SIBO treatment. The study shows that 104 patients diagnosed with SIBO were treated with either herbal antimicrobials or rifaximin (1,200 milligrams) for the period of four weeks and the results found that 46 percent of the patients treated with herbal antimicrobials experienced symptom improvements, when compared with the 34 percent treated with the antibiotic rifaximin. Also, 14 out of the 44 patients who still had SIBO after a course of rifaximin were afterward treated with herbal antimicrobials. 57 percent responded positively to the natural herbal treatment even after failing to feel better from the antibiotics.

7. Oregano Can Help Treat Parasites

One study found that when adults whose stools tested positive for enteric parasites (including Blastocystis hominis which causes digestive distress) supplemented with 600 milligrams of oregano for six weeks many experienced significant gastrointestinal symptoms. There was a "complete disappearance of Entamoeba hartmanni (four cases), Endolimax nana (one case), and Blastocystis hominis in eight cases." Gastrointestinal symptoms improved in seven of the 11 patients who had tested positive for Blastocystis hominis, which tends to cause symptoms like nausea, gas, bloating and abdominal pain.

CHAPTER FOUR

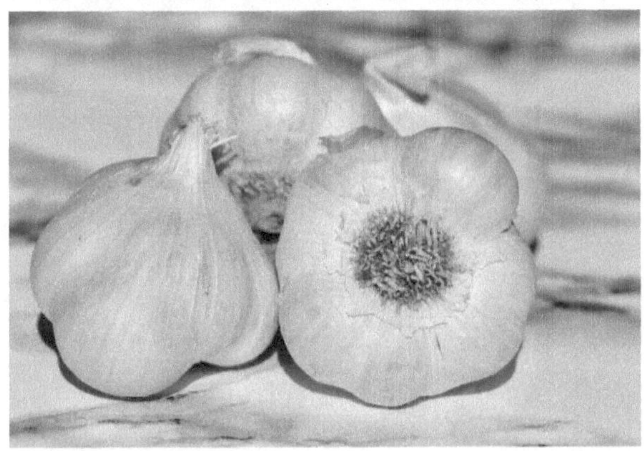

History of Garlic

The word "garlic" comes from Old English garleac, which means "spear leek." As a culinary and medicinal plant, garlic spread in ancient times to the Mediterranean region and beyond. Garlic (Allium sativum) is a plant in the onion family, and it is recognized world-wide for its cooking properties and health effects. Their flavor is unmistakable as just as irreplaceable in sauces, roasting, and as a seasoning for countless dishes. It is high in a sulfur compound called Allicin, which is believed to bring most of the health benefits.

For over 5,000 years garlic has been used as food, medicine, money, an aphrodisiac, and magic potions. It has been revered as an offering fit for the gods and despised as a substance suitable only to be fed male pigs. Garlic has been believed to warded off the evil eye, and was hung over the doors to protect medieval occupants from evil, it gave strength and courage to Greek athletes and warriors, and protected the maidens and pregnant ladies from evil nymphs, and also garlic was rubbed on door frames in order to keep blood thirsty vampires out. Garlic bulbs pendants hung around the neck protected the individual from the sharp horns of a bull, kept away the black plague, and warded off local witches.

Also, garlic has been used for medicinal purposes by more cultures than any other plant product or substance over the years. The first recorded instances of garlic being used for medicinal purposes, was by the Sumerians of Mesopotamia, in the regions of the Tigris and Euphrates rivers.

The consumption of garlic in the United States has tripled since the

1990's, with more people discovering the delightful properties of this bulb. Worldwide there are over 2.5 million acres in garlic cultivation! That's a lot of garlic

History of Garlic in the Far East.

Although garlic was highly regarded as a medicine in eastern cultures, it was never used as a food. Both the Buddhists and Hindus avoided eating garlic. Ancient Indians valued the medicinal properties of garlic and thought it to be an aphrodisiac and was never considered to be suitable food for the upper classes in the society, who detested its strong odor. Garlic was also forbidden by monks, who believed garlic to be a stimulant that aroused sexual passions.

Adolescents, Widows and all those who had taken up a vow, or were fasting, could not eat garlic because of its stimulant quality inherent.

This approach however changed over time with the centuries and period of Muslim rule. Garlic, onion and ginger were, and continue to be, an indispensable part of cuisines of South Asia. In ancient Indian, garlic also has a history of use in Ayurvedic medicine. They used the garlic healing system as a medicinal plant which could warm the body, improve blood circulation, and cure digestive problems.

<u>History of Garlic in Ancient Greek and Roman Life.</u>

Ancient civilizations, such as the Greeks and Romans used garlic to boost strength and prevent diseases. In ancient Rome and Greece, garlic enjoyed a variety of uses, ranging from repelling scorpions down to treating animal bites, bladder infections, curing leprosy and asthma. Garlic was also left out as an offering to the Greek goddess Hectate.

In early Greek military their leaders fed garlic to the troops before battles to give them courage and promise victory. They Greeks also fed their athletes with garlic to give them strength for the Olympic Games. Also, garlic was often used to help heal wounds from battle.

Hippocrates, is who considered the father of western medicine and lived 460 to 370 B.C., was said to have used garlic to treat cancerous tumors. He was said to recommend garlic for pneumonia and other infections, digestive disorders, as well as using it as a diuretic and a substance to ameliorate menstrual flow.

<u>History of Garlic in Egypt.</u>

Archeological findings have shown paintings of garlic, dating back to 3200 B.C, in Egyptian tombs, including the Great Pyramid of Cheops. In Egypt garlic was worshipped and placed clay models of garlic bulbs in the tomb of Tutankhamen. Recently it was discovered that Egyptian papyrus dating from 1,500 B.C. recommends garlic as a cure for more than 22 common ailments, including lack of stamina, heart disease and tumors. It was highly-prized, it was in some cases even used as currency. Although in Egypt garlic was worshipped, they also possess a strong aversion to cooking and eating it. The Egyptian also feed garlic to their slaves building the pyramids just to increase their strength.

Also the ancient Israelites who were in Egypt were fond of garlic long before Moses led them out of the land. In the Mishnah, which is a collection of Jewish traditions incorporated into the Talmud, ancient Hebrew writers refer to themselves as "the garlic eaters." On their way to their Promised Land, the Jews lamented for the absence of garlic, as well as other Egyptian foods.

<u>History of Garlic in Western Cultures.</u>

Garlic has been used as a medication against plagues that struck London in the 17th century and France in the 18th century. The New England, during the colonial period, garlic cloves were used against diseases such rheumatism, smallpox, intestinal worms and those suffering from whooping cough. Louis Pasteur acknowledge the antiseptic properties of garlic in 1858, and Albert Schweitzer used garlic for dysentery.

Garlic was shunned as a food by the western cultures such as England and

America for many years, because of the odor it leaves behind. In the 17th century England, it was considered unfit for ladies and anyone who wished to court them. Garlic was avoided in United States until the 20th century, when a huge influx of immigrants allowed garlic to slowly gain a foothold in the American peninsula.

Garlic became Popular in the 20th Century. Even though it was initially used almost exclusively in ethnic working-class neighborhoods, but by 1940 America had finally embraced garlic, recognizing its value not only a seasoning, but as a major ingredient in recipes.

During the Second World War, garlic was dubbed "Russian penicillin" because garlic was used by the Russian army to fight infections on the battlefield. Garlic was also widely used as an antiseptic to prevent gangrene during both World Wars.

Garlic is today recognized worldwide as an extremely nutritious addition to any diet of choice. There also exist several thousands of papers on the health benefits of garlic that have been published since 1950.

YOUR BODY NEEDS GARLEAC

In the words of ancient Greek physician Hippocrates, often called the father of Western medicine which says "Let food be thy medicine, and medicine be thy food." He was said to have used garlic to treat cancerous tumors and recommend garlic for pneumonia and other infections, digestive disorders, as well as using it as a diuretic and a substance to ameliorate menstrual flow.

As we shall be examining below, raw garlic benefits are plentiful. They are used as an effective form of plant-based medicine in several ways, including the following.

<u>Garlic for Cancer</u>

Bulbous vegetables such as garlic and onions, and their bioactive sulfur compounds are believed to have effects at every stage of cancer formation and affect several biological processes that helps to modify the risk cancer.

The NIH National Cancer Institute has this to say, "Several population studies show an association between increased intake of garlic and reduced risk of certain cancers, including cancers of the stomach, colon, esophagus, pancreas, and breast." This also includes an answer to a very important question: How can garlic act to prevent cancer? They explained that "protective effects from garlic may arise from its antibacterial properties or from its ability to block the formation of cancer-causing substances, halt the activation of cancer-causing substances, enhance

DNA repair, reduce cell proliferation, or induce cell death."

A French research of 345 breast cancer patients proved that increased garlic, onion and fiber intakes were associated with a statistically significant reduction in risk of breast cancer. Also, garlic has been specifically shown to positively affect pancreatic cancer, this is one of the most deadly forms cancer in the world today. The interesting thing is that scientific study has now found that increased in garlic consumption may reduce the risk of developing pancreatic cancer.

A study based on population conducted in the San Francisco Bay area found that pancreatic cancer risk was 54 percent lower in persons who ate larger amounts of garlic and onions compared with those who ate lower amounts. The research also showed that increasing the overall consumption of vegetables and fruits may protect against developing pancreatic cancer.

Also, garlic has shown promises when it comes to cancer treatment. Garlic's organosulfur compounds, including DADS, DATS, ajoene, and S-allylmercaptocysteine (SAMC), have been seen to induce cell cycle arrest when added to cancer cells during in vitro experiments. Adding to these, sulfur compounds have been found to induce apoptosis when added to various cancer cell lines grown in culture. Consuming liquid garlic extract and S-allylcysteine (SAC) orally has also been reported to increase cancer cell death in animal models of oral cancer.

In general, garlic shown clearly some real potential as a cancer-fighting food that should not be discounted or ignored.

Garlic for Diabetes

Garlic has as well proven her ability to help diabetics. Eating garlic has proven to help regulate blood sugar levels, potentially stop or decrease the effects of some diabetes complications, as well as fight infections, encourage circulation and reduce LDL cholesterol.

Research on diabetic rats showed that garlic may be very helpful at improving the general health of diabetics, these includes the mitigation of common diabetic complications like atherosclerosis and nephropathy. These rats, being given a daily extract of raw garlic for seven weeks, significantly had lowered blood sugar level, cholesterol and triglyceride levels. When compared to the control group, these rats receiving raw garlic had 57% less blood sugar level, 40% lower serum cholesterol levels and 35% lower triglycerides. In addition to these, urinary protein levels in garlic-treated rats were 50% lower.

Also, another separate study showed that for type II diabetes patients, garlic significantly improved blood cholesterol levels. Particularly, garlic consumption reduced total cholesterol and LDL cholesterol and moderately raised HDL cholesterol compared to placebo.

Garlic for Heart Disease

Garlic has been generally recognized as both a preventative agent and treatment of many cardiovascular and metabolic diseases, including thrombosis, hyperlipidemia, hypertension, atherosclerosis, and diabetes. According to the Centers for Disease Control and Prevention, heart disease is the No. 1 killer in the United States, and this is closely followed by cancer. A scientific review of experimental and clinical studies of garlic benefits found that, in general, garlic consumption has significant cardio protective effects in both humans as well as animals.

May be the most amazing characteristic of garlic is its ability to help reverse early heart disease by removing plaque buildup in the arteries. In 2016, a randomized, double-blind research published in the Journal of Nutrition that involved 55 patients, between the aged 40 to 75 years, who had been diagnosed with metabolic syndrome. The outcome of the study showed that aged garlic extract effectively reduced plaque in the arteries supplying blood to the heart for patients with metabolic syndrome.

One of the famous researchers, Matthew J. Budoff, M.D., talking on the benefits of garlic said, "This study is another demonstration of the benefits of this supplement in reducing the accumulation of soft plaque and preventing the formation of new plaque in the arteries, which can cause heart disease. We have completed four randomized studies, and they have led us to conclude that Aged Garlic Extract can help slow the progression of atherosclerosis and reverse the early stages of heart disease."

<u>Garlic for High Blood Pressure</u>

A study that looked at the effect of aged garlic extract as an adjunct treatment for people already taking antihypertensive medication yet still having uncontrolled hypertension. An interesting phenomenon of garlic is that has been shown to help control high blood pressure. Garlic has proven itself to be highly effective once again. A research published in the scientific journal Maturitas, assessed 50 people with "uncontrollable" blood pressure. It was discovered that simply taking four capsules of aged garlic extract daily for three months causes the blood pressure to drop by an average of 10 points.

Also, another research published in 2014 showed that garlic has "the potential to lower BP in hypertensive individuals similarly to standard BP medication." Garlic therefore, as in the form of the standardized and highly tolerable aged garlic extract for this study, could work just as well as the prescription for hypertension medications. This research further expressed that garlic's polysulfide promote the opening or widening of blood vessels and, hence, blood pressure reduction.

Garlic for Male and Female Alopecia

In Turkey, a clinical trial was conducted to test the use of garlic to treat baldness. Medical Sciences researchers from Mazandaran

University of Iran tested how garlic gel when applied on the scalp twice a day for three months could affect people taking corticosteroids for hair loss. Alopecia in this context is a common autoimmune skin disease, causing hair loss on the scalp, face and sometimes on other areas of the body.

Researchers found that the use of garlic gel significantly added to the therapeutic efficacy of topical corticosteroid in the treatment of alopecia aerate. Even though the study did not test it expressly, applying garlic-infused coconut oil as a standalone treatment might even be more beneficial as a hair loss remedy because it mitigates the risk of absorbing harmful corticosteroids in the skin.

Garlic for Colds and Infections

Research have shown that certain chemical compounds like allicin which are found in garlic are highly effective at killing countless number of microorganisms that are responsible for some of the most common and rarest infections, including common cold. In a certain study, people took either a placebo or garlic supplements for 12 weeks during cold season. Those that consume garlic were less likely to get a cold, and if peradventure they did get a cold, they are more likely to recover faster than the placebo group. While the placebo group had a much greater likelihood of contracting more than one cold over the 12-week treatment period. The research however attributed to garlic the ability to prevent the common cold virus to its star biologically active component, allicin. Garlic actually might help prevent colds as well as other infections.

Garlic's antiviral, antimicrobial, and antifungal properties can help relieve the common cold as well as other forms of infections. Garlic's active component, allicin in particular is believed to play an important role in this vegetable's antimicrobial powers.

<u>Garlic for Alzheimer's Disease and Dementia</u>

These are diseases that are in form of dementia and can rob people of their ability to think clearly, or remember who they even are and ultimately cannot perform everyday tasks. Garlic contains antioxidants that can support the body's protective mechanisms against oxidative damage that can contribute to these cognitive illnesses.

Talking about Alzheimer's patients, β-amyloid peptide plaques are commonly observed in the central nervous system, and this set of plaque deposits result in the production of reactive oxygen species and cells in the nervous system damage. A research work that was published in the Journal of Neurochemistry found "significant neuro-protective and neuro-rescue properties" of aged garlic extract and their active compound S-allyl-L-cysteine (SAC). The researchers ends their findings by saying that aged garlic extract along with SAC can be used to develop future drugs to treat Alzheimer's disease.

CHAPTER FIVE

EVERY HOME USES ME

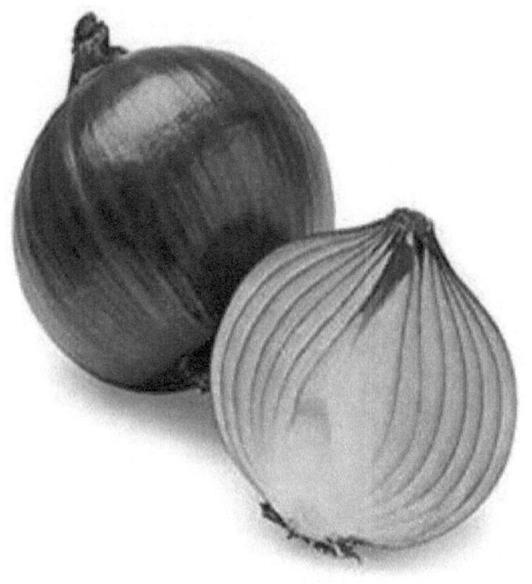

Onion is a staple in most of the known cuisines in the world and a major kitchen ingredients needed and are used to add a colourful texture to your salads, curries, and other kitchen delicacies. Onion does not only adds to the flavour of your food, but it's also has numerous health benefits. Onion according to the book 'Healing Foods' by DK Publishing is a part of the allium family. Onions contains dozens of medicinal chemical compounds with anti-inflammatory and antibacterial actions that protects the body and promote good heart and excellent health. Onions are not only good for kitchen ingredients and for their health benefits, but also for your skin and hair. Onion nutritional composition is quite interesting and it is full of antioxidants and contain a number of sulphur-containing compounds and can be eaten either cooked or raw.

Onions are rich source of antioxidants, minerals, vitamins, and several other vital nutrients like vitamin A, vitamin C and vitamin E which are extremely important for keeping skin ailments at bay. These vitamins present in an onion bulb helps to protect your skin from the harmful effects of ultra-violet rays of the sun.

Onions antioxidants helps to detoxify the body by flushing out toxic substance from our bloodstream. The flushing out of these toxins eventually purifies the skin, thereby preventing the risk of developing any skin ailments.

The components present in onion like quercetin and other sulphur-rich phytochemicals helps to combat free radical damages, as a results can delay the signs of ageing. Also onions has antiseptic, anti-inflammatory and anti-bacterial that may help in preventing breakouts and reducing inflammation. The mineral of content of an onions, especially vitamin C helps in the nourishment of the skin, and making the skin to glow and healthy.

1. Using Onion for Skin and Hair

Onion juice helps to facilitate the formation of keratin that helps your hair to grow. I encourage that you include onion juice to your hair care and skin care regime.

<u>Lemon and Onion Pack</u>

Make ready your onion juice and add some lemon juice in it while mixing together. Use a cotton ball in the prepared solution and apply on your face and neck. Wash it off using cold water when it has dried off. Apply the solution for at least three times a week. This will help protect your from skin developing infections. Why not add onions to your beauty regime and keep your skin healthy and beautiful.

2. Onions Helps Stronger Immunity

Our body mechanism is defended by our immune system and for our body to stay healthy, our immune system must make sure that we do not contract diseases which are caused due to viral infections, fungus, and bacteria. There are many natural ways one can engage to help prevent free radicals from affecting the body and onions is one of them. Onions help us to build a stronger immune system. The presence of vitamin C in an onions is the reason why it is believed to protect our body from several diseases and other viral infections. Also the presence of phytonutrients in onions help the antioxidant properties of an onion to take its full effect.

3. Onions Helps Aids in Antioxidant Production

Vegetables such as onions, broccoli, and cauliflower help our body to produce its own antioxidants. Onions and other of this vegetables is one the best way to help prevent the activities of free radicals. Researches has found that onions help our body produce Glutathione. This Glutathione also helps fight cancerous elements and it is extremely beneficial in maintaining the health of our heart.

4. Onions Helps Prevent Cancer

When Free radicals enters into our body, they cause the growth abnormal cell which leads to the development of cancer. By nature, cancer is a disease that keeps growing if not treated from the onset. Foods can be used to prevent this deadly disease, and reducing its chances through food is the best option. Onions contains Glutathione that helps to fight cancerous elements in our body.

5. Onions Helps Healthy Digestion

Onions is rich in dietary fiber, and this fiber acts as a natural laxative which makes comfortable bowel movements. This fiber helps clean the intestines by removing waste from our body. Also, onions contain saponins which helps to relieve our stomach of cramps and aches.

6. Onions Helps Detoxifying Properties

Detoxing is extremely crucial for our body and has become a popular health trends nowadays. This basically helps the body to flush out several unwanted, toxins and bad cholesterol which is a result of our lack of exercise and bad eating habits.

In keeping our bodies toxin-free, onions is extremely very important. Onions contain amino acids and sulphur-compounds which helps in clearing out our digestive system and also help to expel the harmful toxins from our body.

7. Onions Helps Manage Anaemia

The deficiency of iron in our body could be responsible for anaemia and anaemia is a fatal disease. There are several medications that helps to maintain and balance the levels of haemoglobin in our individual bodies. Using the natural route however helps to prevent the side effects that may be accrue to conventional medication. Onions contain about 0.2mg of iron in every 100 gram and considerably good amount of folate. Folate is often recommended to pregnant women and it's a phytochemical that helps absorb iron to its full potential.

8. Onions Helps Hair Growth

For some certain reasons, sometimes we start losing hair or our hair starts going grey. Several reasons could be responsible for this, it could be due to age, lack of specific nutrients or stress. Consuming potassium and protein rich foods could be very helpful in preventing these complications. Several hair masks can be made with onions to apply, that you can apply directly to your hair and scalp. Onions are not only known for their ability to promote hair growth, but also as a good remedy for dandruff threatening your hair. To use onions for dandruff treatment, mixing your onion juice with yogurt and allow it on your hair for at least half an hour. This can help cleanse your scalp and as well strengthen your hair.

9. Onions Helps in Diabetes Management

If you lead a sedentary lifestyle and eat processed and junk foods diabetes as a chronic disease can hit at anytime. One of the biggest challenge to managing diabetes is the ability to maintain a safe blood sugar level. When onion are consumed raw, it has been found to keep your blood sugar levels in check and also prevent them from getting out of hand.

10. Onions Helps Anti-Aging

The natural antioxidant of an onion is no secret; it helps to increase the internal production of antioxidants in the body. Aging most often is as a result of the accumulation of the harmful substances which the skin absorbs and also by the activities of free radicals. Onions has the antioxidant and detoxifying properties and this to large extent helps slow down the process of aging.

11. Onions Helps Pain Relief

When you scrapped your knee or being stung by a blue bottle or a bee, you can rub a sliced onion on the affected area to help relieve you of pain. This will provide an instant relief from the pain. You can do the same if you have ear irritation, put some few drops of onion juice to a cotton pad and then apply this solution to your ear in order to get rid of the discomfort and pain.

12. Onions Helps Healthy Bones

Onions is also helpful in the treatment of bone loss, onions have been proven to contain growth plate chondrocytes. Inside onions also are compounds that can be very helpful rebuilding of the connective tissue.

13. Onions Helps Anti-fungal and Antimicrobial

Onions does not only prevent viral diseases and infections from entering into our body, but it also help to fight bacteria that are present in our mouths. It is recommended that you chew an onion for 3 minutes in the morning just to get rid of the bacteria that could be found in our mouth.

14. Relieve Cough and Cold Symptoms

Are you suffering from flu virus or a cough, I recommended that you add an onion in hot water when preparing your tea, this will help clear your throat. Also when your Onion juice is added to honey, this can be taken it will help to reduce any swelling in the throat.

www.ingramcontent.com/pod-product-compliance
Lightning Source LLC
Chambersburg PA
CBHW031256250726
48655CB00005B/2244